Loving My Blessings

Removing the Curse of Infertility

Tananda Parson

Loving My Blessings

Removing the Curse of Infertility

TABLE OF CONTENT

So she said to Abram, "The Lord has kept me from having children. Go, sleep with my slave; perhaps I can build a family through her."

Genesis 16:2 NIV

The Lord will always lead you. He will meet the needs of your soul in the dry times and give strength to your body. You will be like a garden that has enough water, like a well of water that never dries up.

Isaiah 58:11 NLT

INTRODUCTION

In 2007, I found myself battling with infertility due to an undiagnosed issue. I could not believe that someone who yearned to have children from such an early age ended up being the one who could not have them. I found myself surrounded by women who were baby-making machines with whom I could only watch and help take care of their little miracles. I decided to trust God in His decision to not allow me to be able to conceive naturally. Not from a lack of trying, of course, but I trusted that His timing was best. This surrendering decision came only after going through some long nights talking with my husbands, several tear-stained pillows, and monthly tantrums when my menstrual cycle would show up unannounced. I stopped buying pregnancy tests because I was making the industry richer and left feeling disappointed each time I received a negative result. If I had children of my own, I do not believe I would have entertained the thought of taking in a stranger's child. Offering them a special nurturing kind of love that would help them get through traumas and separations from their families. I now realize that I was created for such a time as this and have since embraced this calling in my life. During your time of reading, I only ask that you hold onto your seats because my story will be a rollercoaster ride you will not soon forget.

CHAPTER 1
QUESTIONING GOD

I began my journey to motherhood with questions like, "what is wrong with me? Why do I not have any children of my own? Is it not my time yet? Do I need to wait a few more years? Later, those questions drastically changed to, "how am I this close to the age of 40 and have not once known the feeling of a baby kicking in my womb? How have I not experienced childbirth, or the precious bonding of mother and child through breastfeeding?" These are priceless moments I have desired for myself since I was young. I knew that a child would love me unconditionally like no man ever would. This had to be why God saved me from conceiving out of wedlock before I was married. I am not innocent, by any means, but God had to be saving my womb for the many children I would have with my husband. Right? That is why, when I married at the age of 23, I knew that God had heard my prayers and was granting me the desires of my heart. I do have to pause for a moment because I cannot fail to mention the fact that my new husband had met and began entertaining another woman within the first few months of our marriage. But I will dive deeper into that little nugget later in the chapter.

Foolishly, I had my baby plans all mapped out like I was in control of my life. I now know what it means when the Bible says, "you can make plans, but the Lord's purpose will prevail." I wanted to be and had assured myself that I would be done birthing babies by the age of 25. Somehow, I was convinced that I would certainly give birth to twins so that my womb retired according to my timeline. This plan was not very reasonable because there were not any twins genetically in my bloodline that I was aware of. Why did I think I could manipulate my eggs into doing something that was not written into my DNA code? I had been on birth control since I was sixteen and I had no idea if I was even capable of getting pregnant. But here I was. A woman with all the right parts. How hard could it be to conceive? I would soon find out. This double pregnancy would have to be a miracle that only God could perform. He heard my prayers, and I was somewhat faithful, so I prayed to God like He was my personal genie. Thinking that He had to grant my wishes, but I learned that wish-granting was far from the attributes of God. As you will read, my story will reveal God's true nature of love, patience, kindness, and giving.

Now that we have gotten that established, let's jump right into the beginning of my story.

I married my husband in early spring on a beautiful sunny day. I was an hour late to my own nuptials, but it was not because I had hesitations. I was running late due to working the overnight shift. In addition, I also had numerous last-minute errands that needed to be completed to make my big day perfect after only a couple hours of sleep. I have no clue what my soon-to-be husband was doing or why he was unavailable to assist but I got the tasks done. And there he was standing at the altar when I walked down the aisle toward him. It was a day to remember that we happily celebrated with close family and friends. We also had a night he would never forget. That's because I slept through it. There was absolutely no consummation on our wedding night. My body was fatigued due to lack of sleep, and I'd ignored feeling unwell because I was so focused on the wedding. Once the adrenaline of the day wore off, the sickness attacked me hard and all I could do was crawl into bed. He understood that I was not rejecting him. I just physically could not perform. However, as a new bride, I did not want to start our marriage out by neglecting my new husband, so I did make up for it in a couple of days.

Before we wed, my husband had decided to join the military to earn a living for his new family. This meant he would ship out to boot camp a week after we said I DO, leaving me home alone for almost a year. I did not see him again until he graduated from basic training six months later and then again three months later, after he had reached his first duty station. This was not the married life I had anticipated. I figured we would be well on our way to settling into married life and discussing baby names by now. However, due to extended time in training, he was sent ahead to a duty station six states away from home without me. His wife! Needless to say, I was excited when I received news that I could finally join him and get our life started together. I began searching online for places to live since this would be my first time living in a different state. I was nervous and wanted to do as much research as possible about the city I would soon be calling home. Little did I know, he was doing a little recognizance of his own, but we will get to that.

I was able to join him at his new duty station by the end of the same year we got married. I thought this was the perfect time to reunite and start our life together as the current year ended and a new year began. He returned home to pack up and relocate his blushing bride after the Christmas holiday. We made the twenty-four-hour trip by car with a few hiccups that left us spending New Year's Eve stranded in a hotel room a few states away from our intended destination. This delay turned our trip into more of a seventy-two-hour adventure. Nevertheless, once we were back on the road, we continued to the Lone Star State. Arriving around the crack of dawn, we moved our belongings into our new apartment, and married life finally began for us. I made sure my husband had three meals a day, he was pleased in the bedroom, and I was available to handle his wants and needs. I performed all the typical wifely duties like cooking, cleaning, and laundry. I already knew I would be happy in my new role as a wife and mother because it was all I ever wanted to do.

I found a job within the first couple of months to ensure we were financially set. I was able to work at a job that fulfilled me, come home to the love of my life, and fix all the delicious recipes I had seen my mom cook for my dad when I was growing up. I had everything I wanted, and it showed when I started gaining happy weight. Now, I was fine with the weight gain if he was. I was still the beautiful woman he had married, and I made sure she was always packaged well. I had only been in this role for a short time but when we came upon our one-year anniversary, our relationship began to shift in a different direction. We made plans to get away and celebrate since we had not had an official honeymoon. It was going to be so wonderful having him all to myself. No jobs to report to, no alarm clocks to force us awake. Just him and I, spending quality time together. While away, we did some mountain climbing, visited new restaurants, and explored a little sightseeing while enjoying each other's company. It was an awesome trip. We were happy. I also had the photos to prove it just in case anyone asked. We returned home from our trip, both tired and ready to call it a night. Yet right before he got in bed, he felt the need to make a late-night phone call, to his mother, in the spare bedroom, with the door closed. This sparked some suspicions, but I remained silent. "Why did he need to leave the room to call his mother? Was he planning a surprise? Did I do something wrong?" My mind was racing with questions. He came back and innocently joined me in bed, but I could not sleep. Luckily for me, he was a heavy sleeper and had already drifted off. I left the bed and saw that he had plugged his phone up to charge in the kitchen. I wondered why he felt the need to do that? Since he did leave it unattended, I had the perfect opportunity to see if he had indeed called his mother. I grabbed his phone and began searching. It was not long before I found text messages from a woman who was concerned because she had not heard from him for a few days. I took the liberty of responding to her inquiry for him since I did not want her to be worried.

"I mean, what was I supposed to do? Leave her wondering?"

She was surprised when I told her she had not heard from him because we had just returned home from celebrating our first anniversary. It wasn't long before I realized that the woman, I was speaking with was oblivious to the fact that MY husband was a married man. Apparently, she and my husband started communicating while we were separated for those few short months, and he had been lying to both of us this entire time. I was furious! She had the nerve to apologize and wish me luck in my marriage. She obviously thought I needed it with the messy situation I now found myself in. I waited a couple of days to confront him, and he blatantly lied to my face. Stating that the number in his phone belonged to one of his homeboys. He thought this was the smartest response because the contact information was saved under just initials. "How stupid did he think I was?" After some probing and nagging from me, he finally admitted that she was a part of his life and expressed that he would handle it. I trusted him to do just that. I did not tell him that I had already spoken with her but simply told him to get rid of his girlfriend. I believed he would. After all, we were married, and he said he loved me. I will admit that I may have been a little naïve back then.

We both wanted a big family, so we had already quit using birth control early in the marriage to immediately start trying to conceive. However, having a mistress was not a part of the plan. I did not want to get pregnant just to be divorced and raise children on my own. Between him coming and going on work missions, we saw less of each other. During this time, we also kept trying to conceive but with no success. Failing to hit the mark left me questioning my womanhood, the state of my marriage, and left him with wandering eyes. It seems the messy situation I had previously found myself in had only gone away temporarily. Imagine my surprise when I found out months later, he was still communicating with the same woman.

CHAPTER 2
ACCEPTING MY LIFE

Honestly, I was hurt after learning that he was still being unfaithful and slightly perturbed that the other woman along with him, had decided that my marriage was unvaluable. How could she go against the woman code? I thought we had parted ways in a solidarity that said she had no desire to mess up our happy home. More importantly, how could he treat me this way? Had he lost his mind? He obviously had forgotten that I had left my family, friends, and everything I knew to come to be with him. How dare he take advantage of me? I cried and vented to my best friend and his sister who also could not believe he would do this to me. No one, including me, saw this coming. Definitely not within the first two years of us being married. I did not sign up for this type of marriage, especially since I was doing everything I knew how, to be a good wife to him.

After speaking with his sister, who was just as upset as I was, I concocted a plan to truly get his attention. She agreed that he needed to be taught a lesson and would not say a word to him about my plan. I fixed dinner like I normally would and waited for him to come home from work. We spent the evening watching tv while he relaxed and then eventually went to bed. The next morning, I fixed him a hot breakfast before he left for work and while he was gone, I prepared his lunch and cleaned the house. I then sat down and wrote him a "Dear John" letter admitting to him that I knew he was still engaging with another woman. I expressed that this is not the married life I had signed up for and as a result, I was leaving him. I reminded him that I had left my family, friends, and everything familiar to start a life with him because he had chosen to join the military. That well thought out decision came so that he could ensure he would be a good provider for our family. Our family. Not for me, him, and a mistress. I wrote how I was a faithful wife, caring for his every need and I did not deserve to be treated this way. I was not someone he could easily just toss aside because of immaturity and irresponsibility. I finally told him that I had hired movers to come to get my belongings from the house. This part was untrue and a bit extreme, but I wanted him to fully understand the possibility that I would not be returning to live a life with a man who lied to my face over and over.

Once I was done pouring my frustrations out on paper, I placed the handwritten letter in an envelope and tucked it away. He would be home shortly on his lunch break so, to ensure that he did not suspect a thing, I packed his lunch to-go and waited for him in my usual spot at the front door. When he arrived, I kissed him lovingly, gave him a cool drink, then led him into the bedroom and had sex with my lying cheating husband for the last time. He returned to work with his lunchbox and a smile on his face, while I placed the sealed envelope on the same pillow, where he had just laid his head. I left several hours later and went to work knowing he would come home, find the letter, and surely be surprised that his loving wife had just left him.

Still, our story does not end there.

My husband returned home from work and found the letter. He immediately raced to my job within the same hour to profess his undying love and beg me not to leave him. I purposefully left him sitting in the lobby for about an hour while I continued to work. During that time, I could overhear him talking to his mother, and I could only imagine her telling him how stupid he was to cheat on a good woman. Offering suggestions as to how he could make things right. Feeling defeated, he attempted a grand gesture by changing his phone number so that the other woman could not call him anymore.

When we finally sat down together to talk about the issue, he even shed a few tears to prove he would never do it again. I reasoned that he could just as easily call her if he got the urge again, but that's not the point. I asked him why he felt the need to still be talking to other women if he had chosen to get married. His answer was that he was confused and still thinking like a bachelor. I exclaimed that we had been living together under the same roof for a few months as husband and wife according to the rings and vows we exchanged a little over year before. He stated that because we had lived apart for almost the entire first year of marriage he didn't "feel" married. This should have been a red flag, but I chose to ignore it and give him another chance. After all, he was my husband and neither of us believed in divorce because we both grew up in church. I admitted to him that he was not the only one being pursued by the opposite sex, however, I chose to honor my wedding vows even though we were separated. Besides, my faith in God was a little shaky back then and my trust level did not allow me to even think about what living a divorced life would be like. I wanted to be married and raise children with the same man just like my parents. They had been married for over 25 years and I wanted the same longevity in my marriage. I could not picture myself jumping back in the dating pool looking for another person to love me forever. So, I accepted his apology, with some stipulations, and things went back to normal married life, or so I thought.

We continued dreaming about what our children would look like and trying to get pregnant with no success. We tried to see the brighter side of not having children, whereas we could come and go as we pleased at a moment's notice without having to find a babysitter. However, since he was the only male child, he needed to have a son to carry on his name and bloodline. This was proving to be a not so easy task and now I discovered I had a new problem to add to the plate. Suffering silently from depression left little room for any other joys in my life except the wonderful taste of food. And I could always find good food to keep me company. I did not recall until much later that as a child I would sneak and take food out of the kitchen to eat it in secret. Not because I was hungry, but because I just really liked the taste of food and it never rejected me. That habit clearly remembered me and was taking full control of my life now that I was responsible for feeding myself. I kept a smile on my face and went about life, but I ate to cope and gained weight that far surpassed any scale number that I had previously known. Yes, my clothes were a little tighter, but I could still squeeze into them, so I didn't see the weight creeping on.

This was much more than just happy fat. My friends that were around me did not seem to notice or did not have the heart to point out that I was getting bigger. I was frustrated and tired of waiting for my miracle, so I did what I knew how to do. I ate my feelings. Every last one of them. Although I was Auntie to all my friend's kids and was blessed to be an integral part of their lives, there was still this unfulfilled longing to have children of my own. To see my pregnant belly when I looked in the mirror. To have other mothers give me advice on how to raise a brand-new baby. To be able to finally give my parents a grandchild. The list went on and on. But how could I express this out loud without sounding selfish and ungrateful? I wanted children and I wanted them now! It was not until I saw a photo of myself sitting with those same friends one day that I realized I had gained an immense amount of weight, and this was probably contributing to my infertility as well. I was always out eating with them so that I would not be alone through my husband's deployments and field training. Whether it was breakfast, lunch, brunch, or dinner, I was available to go out, even if I had just eaten. But they didn't need to know that. I became the go-to person for meal companionship and spent a lot of our savings on restaurants and fast food. Nonetheless, after seeing that photo, I was determined to lose that weight before my husband came home. Yes, we were apart, yet again, for a year while he was deployed. But when he returned, I did not want there to be any reason that he would find me undesirable or have any obstacles that could hinder me from getting pregnant this time around. I was in school at the time and a classmate recommended I go see a weight loss specialist because they had helped her through her weight loss journey. I got the information and went to the weight loss center to seek help with losing the excess weight. I knew I could not do it on my own because food was too tempting, and it was the only thing currently making me happy. I was embarrassed during my initial consultation to learn that I was almost 270 pounds, and nobody had said a word about it. However, by sticking to their strict eating plan, and regimen, I successfully lost thirty pounds! I surprised myself seeing how I could achieve that goal by having some self-control over the things I was eating. I felt sexy and empowered again.

I knew the weight loss would certainly help me get pregnant since this was one of the suggestions that were made by my physician. This had to work! Once my husband returned home, he was shocked to see the new me. I was back down to the scale number from my college days when he and I first met. He had no clue that I had loss so much weight because I had stopped sending him pictures of me while he was deployed. I secretly, did not want to disappoint him if I had failed, so I kept the weight loss a surprise. With no time to waste, we immediately resumed trying to have a baby. My husband did not share with me how he felt about us not being able to get pregnant, but I could tell the pressure was affecting him. He started secretly smoking cigarettes at work, which was disappointing because nicotine can also lower sperm count. We did not need any more negative hits in this area. They say practice makes perfect, so we practiced a lot, but the lie detector test determined that was a lie. With no successful conception this time, we were forced to turn to fertility experts and doctors. After rounds of several very invasive tests that determined the viability of my ovaries and fallopian tubes, they tested him for his sperm count and started me on hormone injections to kick my body into ovulation. But it seemed, the odds were just not working in our favor. The doctors were baffled because it was determined that there was absolutely no reason why I could not or had not conceived yet. This was good news that somehow frustrated me even more. Why was God not allowing me to get pregnant? Why was I not able to have all the children we had dreamed about? Why God? Why?

CHAPTER 3

TO ADOPT OR NOT TO ADOPT

After a couple years of still not getting pregnant, we started to throw around the option of adoption. I could not understand how my biological mother had four kids back-to-back, plus another one years later, and I could not conceive just one. Even my biological grandmother had given birth to five or six children and all of them have children and grandchildren. What was wrong with me? My husband did not have any previous children either, so he wondered if he could be contributing to our infertility issues as well. However, we wanted to have a baby that looked like us, so we kept trying, to no avail. We planned sex around his work schedule to ensure we did not miss even one opportunity to catch the egg during ovulation. The only issue was that from the time I was a teen, my menstrual cycles were irregular, which made the timing of ovulation hard to pinpoint.

In most cases, when a woman does not have her menstruation, she might be ovulating or pregnant. In my case, I never knew when I could be ovulating, which is the first step to trying to get pregnant. I extensively researched what sexual positions would result in pregnancy. I investigated Karma Sutra and seriously considered using the turkey basting method to see if we could hit the jackpot. I was desperate for anything that would guarantee we got pregnant. Our sex life transitioned from spontaneous and fun to exhausting and stressful.

Every year went by with no success, and I felt more and more like a failure, so I became an entrepreneur to stay busy. I had to try to do something right. First, I provided childcare for friends and family, and then I opened my own catering business. Although, around year four or five of marriage, I can remember being asked to take in a set of family twins that were soon to be born. I thought, well, maybe this is the way God wants us to begin our family. He knew that I desired to have twins, so this had to be the miracle answer to my prayers! I fasted and prayed for the twins to come to us after they were born, but we never heard anything else from the family member. I waited and waited, but it was as if they had changed their minds but were too afraid to tell us. I had already purchased baby clothing, picked out baby names, and looked at crib accessories. I felt like Hannah crying out to God in the temple once again because my womb was still empty. This had to be His fault! Was God teaching me a lesson? Did I do something that made me undeserving of being a mother?

I was devastated yet again and finally decided that adoption would be the solution to my fertility issues. Since I, myself, had been adopted, I was not totally opposed to the idea. I just thought that I would always birth my own children. Coincidentally, as only God could have orchestrated it, my adoptive mother and my stories are somewhat similar. Unlike us, she and my dad were able to conceive but was unable to carry to term and miscarried twice. They were unable to have children of their own for the first seven years of marriage.

However, God saw fit to bless her with a close relative's two-week-old infant, that she would adopt within six months, thus starting her adoption journey. A few months later, she would receive a call from a friend about my two brothers and me. We were being displayed on the evening news during an adoption segment and it was their last plea to find someone willing to adopt three kids under the age of four. It was urgent that someone came forward because we were on the verge of being split up in hopes that we could be easily adopted as a single child versus a package of three. Of course, I did not know this at the time, but my Granny had instilled in her a sense of family and togetherness that ensured that no matter the hardships or struggles they faced, the family would stay together. Remembering my granny's determination, my mom made it her mission to contact The Department of Social Services to inquire about our whereabouts. After discussing it over with my father they started the process to see how they could go about adopting us. Now, we had been in foster care for over a year by that time and our biological family nor relatives had come forward to take custody of us.

Luckily, we had already been taken in by a loving older couple who fostered us until we were adopted by my parents. I was told that my biological mother did come to visit with us during that time. However, I was too young to remember so the origin of my adoption story is unclear. This includes the missing details of why we were removed from our mother's residence, how we ended up in the custody of Child Protective Services, and why we were never returned home. What I can say with conviction is, I am extremely grateful to have been adopted into a family that wanted me and my siblings. What I have learned in the past few years is that being chosen by someone who wants you does not negate or erase the rejection and insecurity you experience because of the actions and choices of the people who should have wanted you. Who should have chosen you. These feelings were amplified after the one and only conversation I've ever had with my biological father about 15 years ago. He could not offer an acceptable reason for his absence or a valid excuse as to why he didn't choose us. I am convinced that he walked away from his four children and selfishly made the decision to not look back. I can also say that my biological mother desired to take care of us because of her love for us but could not make the necessary decisions or actions needed to keep all of us in her care. She was able to keep one child because she was pregnant at the time we were put into foster care. I cannot speak for my brothers, but I can say that after looking back at the bits and pieces of scraps I've been told about the first couple of years of my life, it sometimes leaves me feeling as if I was just thrown away or traded in for a newer model or that I was not worthy enough for them to choose me. But thank God for the option of adoption. It changed the whole trajectory of my life and set me right where I am today. I would not have the strength to keep going if it was not instilled into me by my strong adoptive mother.

So, like I said, this option was somewhat familiar and was certain to be our last chance to become parents. Our last hope to create the family we wanted. I just knew in my heart that if we had children, our marriage would become stronger and would last forever. I was sadly mistaken.

CHAPTER 4

OPENING MY HEART AND HOME

In the meantime, my little sister, from my biological mother, had come to visit, so I had a little bit of a distraction. In hindsight, her presence got me through the next couple years of marriage since I did not have time to dwell on my unhappiness while taking care of her. We never started the process of adoption because I became busy with raising my sister. I had no clue that my little sister would become my first unofficial foster child. First off, I did not meet her until she was the age of 15, so our relationship started off unique. We could not spend a lot of time getting to know one another due to my work schedule and her still being in high school with no driver's license or vehicle. The relationship between my birth mom and I was still new and strained, which made the phone conversations with my little sister just as awkward. I realized that our conversations were being monitored, so my best friend and I made plans to celebrate her birthday with a Sweet 16 slumber party. This party helped to get her out of the house for a whole weekend. Just from our brief phone conversations, I could see she needed to get a taste of freedom as a young teenager. As our relationship grew closer, I soon found out that her parents were sheltering her way too much and she was suffering from a childhood trauma of her own.

Surprisingly, she asked to come to visit me one summer after she had turned 17. I was now living in another state, so we had not seen each other in a few months. I convinced her parents to let her come visit, but it was disastrous from the beginning. She missed her connecting flight causing me to drive an additional hour to meet her plane. We then had to search for her luggage that unfortunately got lost in transition. After finally getting back home to get her settled, I was excited to begin our sisterhood bonding time, but that had to wait. When we unpacked her large suitcase, to my surprise, it was filled with too small clothing that had to be replaced immediately. She later revealed that she had not seen a dentist in years when I questioned her hygiene routine, and please do not get me started on her child-like behavior. As we got into a daily routine, I was taken aback at how pre-teen her thinking was and how trips to the Dollar Tree excited her like a toddler on Christmas.

Consequently, she grew up by leaps and bounds over that summer, learning about hygiene, boys, God, faith, laundry, and whatever else her aunties could teach her. She even had her first trip to the optometrist. Discovering that her view of the world had been blurred for majority of her life. After she received her brand-new glasses, you would think she had hit the lottery.

She kept me company that summer, and unbeknownst to her, she also helped me survive my husband's last deployment. She thrived so much so, that she made the decision to remain in my care and finish out her high school senior year living with me. Afterward, she became an independent young adult with real goals. Learning to drive and choosing a military career path straight out of high school was a huge milestone for her. I remember being a nervous parent watching her go on her first date with a respectable young man whom I was glad she could spend time with. I was a proud mama. Never did I accuse our mother of being a horrible role model, but it was quite evident that my sister had not learned enough to make it in the adult world until she came to live with me. Without financial assistance from her parents, it taught me to love and care for her as if she were my own child. This was the first lesson I was grateful to have learned before entering the world of Child Protective Services and Foster Care. I could not base the way I cared for children on the dollar amount attached to the child. It did not cost me anything to love a child wholeheartedly.

By that time, my husband and I had been married for about four years. We decided to give up our home to save money, while he was away training for a new military occupational specialty. Things did not work out the way we planned, and we became homeless due to unforeseen circumstances. After bouncing from house to house, we found ourselves sleeping in our friend's spare bedroom until we got back on our feet. My sister had graduated high school and left for boot camp with the United States Air Force by this time. While she was away, we decided to buy a house to be settled in before she returned. Unfortunately, she was medically discharged after an extended time in training due to an injury, so she also had to move into our friend's house unexpectedly. Imagine adding a family of three into a home that already had a family of seven and sometimes eleven during the summer months. We were extremely grateful that they were kind enough to accept us into their spacious home. This allowed us the time and opportunity to build our own home instead to design it the way we wanted. Once my sister returned and was settled, she started working locally and was able to purchase her first car all on her own, with a little help from one of her uncles. We were all so excited to see the joy she had when she showed off her new set of car keys. Though she did not advance to the military career she desired, she did have time to positively influence those training alongside her with her contagious laugh and witty personality. She left a lasting impression on all who met her and was sad to leave her battle buddies behind. But she was glad to be back at home with her family.

My sister became active in the church and gave her life to Christ. It was so beautiful watching her flourish into a confident young woman. She finally mustered up the courage to join the worship team after being afraid for months to sing in a mic. I can still remember her little two-step dances as she sang along to the music in her own little world. She was the happiest she had ever been. Sadly, my little sister did not live to see the age of 20. It was one night during a random thunderstorm that we lost her. Floodwaters swept her sports car off the road into a ravine on her drive home from work. I can remember being on pins and needles as we searched well into the midnight hour, hoping that the witness who claimed to have seen her car slide off the road was mistaken. He was not. After searching across the city, we circled back and sat in a parked SUV a few feet away from the scene of the incident all night. Holding cups of coffee that had once been piping hot but were now a lukewarm weight in our hands. Just waiting and watching the area that had been blocked off by police cars, slowly become more visible as the new day dawned. It was just after dawn before the Search and Rescue's Dive Team were able to jump into the ravine to retrieve her from her car. Hearing them break the car window, knowing what they were doing at that very moment, had me holding my breath, praying for a miracle. The wait was excruciating, and it is nothing I ever want to experience again. I don't know what was worse. Bracing myself as the police chief walked toward me to tell me what I already knew or having to identify her body, with family and friends looking on in the distance hoping it wasn't her.

Unfortunately, it was my little sister who they had pulled out of the water. The one who I had the privilege of seeing grow up right before my eyes. The one who I had fearlessly taught to drive her very first car. The one who I had just helped pick out the beautiful yellow blouse she wore for work the day before. The same blouse that was now dirty and dingy from sitting in the murky water all night. They saw me looking at the bruises on her hand and explained that it was a sign that she was fighting to get out of the car. She was not a quitter and had fought until the end. Without warning, my little sister was gone.

There was nothing that could have prepared me for the unfamiliar pain that tore through me as my world was crushed. I smiled lovingly at her peaceful face, held my head up, and walked away. I could not face the coroner as he zipped up the body bag and placed her in the dark once more. No one knew what to say as they were as shocked as I was. My husband and I went home to deliver the devastating news by phone, first to my parents, and then to hers, because I did not have the strength to do it alone. My parents were shocked and flew in immediately to support and comfort me during this difficult time while I planned her funeral celebration. Now, a few weeks prior to this incident we had almost completed our home building project, but that contract had fell through and we lost the beautiful home we built for the three of us. However, being here at my friend's house, everywhere I turned reminded me of my sister, so I pleaded with my husband that we needed to move out immediately. We found a home for rent within days after her death and moved in. We had plenty of space in our new home, so we invited her parents to fly in and stay with us during this time. Imagine my surprise when her parents chose not to come. Instead, they decided to have her body shipped back home where they lived and planned their own funeral. I was heartbroken, to say the least, but there was nothing I could do since, biologically, and legally, they were her parents.

I did not let their decision deter me from celebrating the life of my amazing sister. We still had our own service in her memory, singing her favorite songs, and reminiscing about her unforgettable dancing. Her favorite gospel singer and recent winner of Sunday's Best, Le'Andria Johnson, also flew in and made a special appearance ending the celebration on a high note. Days after the funeral, I was now faced with the daunting task of cleaning out her belongings that still occupied my friend's front office. It had become her temporary bedroom while we built our new home with a new bedroom, she had already picked out. Her death was such an unexpected punch in the gut and at times, it was hard for me to even breathe. I did not know how to move forward and just continue living life without her. This was also my first experience having to grieve the loss of a child that I did not birth, so I did not know how to process my feelings. Although selfishly, I wished none of this had happened and thought often, "if only she had taken a different route." The only peace I was able to have in the situation was knowing that she was with God. That same peace is what carries me every time I think about my baby sister. I can laugh about the dance parties we had, the midnight sister talks, and her transition from a silly child into a young God-fearing Christian woman. The only regret that I have is that her parents and family back home did not get the chance to know this wonderful young woman she had become in such a short time. She is my angel who taught me to love every child that comes through my home as if they were my own.

A year later, some of our church members offered to hold a memorial celebration where she passed away in her honor. Because of the impact she had on all our lives; I knew this was important for everyone. It was a tough year following her death and this memorial was something I was looking forward to. However, my husband forbade it and did not allow it to take place stating, "she's not there anymore so we're not celebrating where she died." I believe that choice was the last straw for me internally concerning my marriage. It left me wondering whether this was another sign that we should not be together. It seemed like the signs were adding up.

As I stated before, I did not believe in divorce and did not think it was an option because my parents were still married after 30 plus years. Although I had seen a few of my relative's relationships end, I did not want to believe that my marriage could possibly be over, so I threw myself into my work. Cooking and catering for local engagements and gatherings on the weekends and still working my full-time job during the week. I did this for the next few years with the help of friends and family. My husband had been discharged from the military and decided to further his education by this time, so he was home more often. I realized I was working extremely hard with minimal support from him which made it harder to be successful due to burnout. I recognized that he now had more time to help me, but I did not want to have to beg my husband for help when he could clearly see it was needed. I may have been a little stubborn back then, but I was also beginning to see this man in a whole new light. And I was totally over it. I felt he was very self-serving and did not reciprocate the same support I gave him unless it was beneficial to him. This of course was partly my fault because I allowed it to continue for so long. After concluding in my mind that our relationship was not getting better, and sadly we weren't having kids, I blurted out my frustrations to him one Sunday after church in the Sonic parking lot. He could sense that something was bothering me because I wasn't eating my food and he knew I loved Sonic onion rings! So, he poked and prodded until I finally exclaimed that I was unhappy in our marriage, I felt like we were going in different directions, and I wanted a divorce. He was extremely surprised by my confession and looked at me like I had sprouted two heads. He could not seem to understand how I could not be satisfied with our relationship. To prove my point, I could have explained how our friends were there for me emotionally when he couldn't even see I was hurting. Or how our marriage was geared more towards what he wanted verses what was best for us. I could have easily listed every time he had a grand idea that cost us money and time we could never get back after it failed, like when we were homeless. Also, how he had to be in the spotlight whenever we were around other people. But I simply explained how I needed someone who supported my dreams and goals because they wanted the both of us to succeed. Someone who allowed me room to be myself and a safe space to not be ok when I really wasn't ok. And someone who loved me the way I desired to be loved. The fact that he was unaware of how I felt let me know that I hid my disappointment very well. I had kept quiet for too long or he had stopped paying attention to his wife. Either way, after seeking spiritual guidance, attempting to compromise, and relapse in judgment, our marriage would end in divorce after nine and a half years of pretending we were happy.

He remarried within six months of our divorce becoming final as if our life together was easily replaceable. That news was a slap in the face and my suspicions of another woman were proven to be true. They would conceive within two or three years of marriage further letting me know that I was the issue. Either my womb decided to reject his seed, or it was not in the plan of God that I should be attached to him for another eighteen years. Nevertheless, my journey involving him stopped there.

CHAPTER 5

STARTING OVER AGAIN

As a newly appointed single woman, I had plenty of time to myself. My marriage ending was a surprise to everyone because we looked like we were happy for so long. Going through the divorce process I questioned if I had made the right decision because he was not physically abusing me or cheating that I was aware of at the time. In the end, I concluded that we should have gone to counseling early on in our marriage to discover how we could prosper as a married couple and truly stay committed to one another. However, it was emotionally draining me to pretend like he was making me happy, and we were past the point where counseling was going to rescue us. And to be honest, he didn't put forth a real fight for us even with knowing that a divorce was possibly ahead. I guess that's because he already had a plan b. I did not realize at the time that I shouldn't have been depending on him to make me happy anyway and the real disappointing truth is that I should have waited to get married. I was scarred and damaged from men in my past that had used me for their own selfish reasons, and I chose to marry because he had shown me something slightly different while we were dating. Apparently, that was a lie too. He only told me what I wanted to hear but he wasn't much different from the others. After I found out he was swiftly engaged to another woman before the ink could dry on our divorce papers, I realized that I needed time to heal and move on. Time to wallow in self-pity, time to question why I let my marriage go, and time to figure out what I was going to do next. While I was trying to figure out what to do with my life, a sister-friend convinced me to go through a Foster Care training class to become a foster parent. I was not at all interested in the beginning because I did not desire to be a single parent. Honestly, I only signed up because I had more free time now and a lot of empty space in my new home to care for a child. I attended the weekly training sessions and became more interested. When they asked what age range I was looking for, I immediately knew I wanted a baby, but I chose an age range of zero to six years old just in case there were no newborns available. It felt very much like choosing a product from some catalog, but I had to remember that these were actual lives.

The training was very informative and eye-opening. It covered topics like how to take care of children who had been through trauma and ways to reassure children that they were in a safe place. We discussed, what to do if the child placed in your home rejects you, and what constitutes discipline versus what is deemed abuse. This particular discussion took me back to my childhood. I knew that a lot of disciplinary tactics used when I was a child would now be considered abuse. This challenge would require me to be strategic in my parenting and think outside of the box when it came to discipline. When they got to the topic of financial compensation, I was taken aback that it was completely normal to become a foster parent to supplement your income. I thought it was strangely selfish that people would receive children in their homes just for the money.

I had dived into this new venture headfirst with minimum knowledge of how the foster care system worked. I only knew that I wanted a baby, and it seems, this route was how I was going to get one. I received my certificate for completing the training and thought that I would immediately receive a baby. It did not work that way. The process outside of the classroom training was more invasive and required me to do extra work, but I was willing. I had to make some adjustments in my home to make sure that it was safe for a child's arrival. Strangers came out to inspect my home, ensuring I had a fire extinguisher, a fire escape plan, and both chemicals and medication were locked away. Oddly, they also checked for food and running water. Are these not essential for anyone's home? Why did they feel the need to invade my privacy by checking my refrigerator and pantry or looking in my personal bedroom? The spare bedroom was set up with beds and children's toys. I felt this was what was most important to look for. Although I was a bit nervous to become a licensed foster parent, I was also excited to receive a new addition to my home and could not wait for his or her arrival. But waiting is exactly what I did.

For almost a whole year.

During that year-long wait, I was on an emotional rollercoaster. Following my divorce, I had to learn how to live alone again which was a major struggle for me. My home was void of laughter, love, energy, and me. I was barely there. I quit my job, joined a gym, swiped left on dating sites, and spent a lot of my time sleeping on other people's couches just so that I did not have to be alone with my depressing thoughts. I was lonely and not fit to be anyone's mother in this state of mind. There was still a mix of emotions teetering between the excitement of possibly adopting and being terrified of raising kids alone. My life was not supposed to go this way. Eventually, my home was licensed and ready to receive children. Within hours of my home being approved and licensed, I received the call that a child needed placement. Although this was not my desired plan for parenting, it looked like being a single parent was what I would be doing whether I was ready or not.

I received a five-year-old little girl who just needed a home until her parents were able to find suitable living arrangements and complete a family plan set in place by the courts. She was the sweetest little girl, and it snapped me out of my funk. I could not have asked for a better first placement and I came to love her as if she were my own. I thought that if this was how the kids were going to be, it should not be difficult to find one I could adopt. We got into a rhythm that worked for us and instantly became a family. Since she was school-aged and very active, my life as a single parent was kicked into gear. She started Kindergarten, joined a community cheerleader squad, and fit right in with my family and friends. We traveled to visit my family back home and they fell in love with her as quickly as I did. However, she only resided with me for about ten months before she was reunited with her family, leaving me with a new little girl who had been placed with us a few weeks prior. We were so sad to see her go but was hopeful that her parents had done the necessary work to keep her safe from now on. Even though she was not the newborn that I initially desired, we formed an unbreakable bond. Given the opportunity, I would have adopted her without question.

I recalled from the training class that once you passed the six-month mark, adoption became an option that was open for discussion. However, family reunification is always the first choice of the court if it is a viable solution. Her leaving left a void in my heart and in the home. This emptiness was felt by me and the new three-year-old who had already been titled her "sister." This left me and the new little girl, who was of different ethnicity, a chance to get acquainted. The new child proved to be more of a challenge in the beginning. I can recall walking through the house one day looking for her because she was not in her bed. I went into the kitchen and saw she had climbed up onto the counter looking for food. Another day I walked in to find her sitting on the floor with the refrigerator door open, eating cheese. Judging by her actions, it was clear, she spent a lot of time alone, learning to get food the best way she could. She did not speak much English and would randomly scream when she could not clearly communicate or get what she wanted.

Imagine being in the middle of the store where she falls out on the floor, throwing a massive tantrum that included high-pitched screaming. This got everyone's attention and embarrassed me. As I got to know her better, I suspected that she had some undiagnosed autistic tendencies. However, I would fall in love with this little girl, and she would be the first child to call me "mommy." There were a lot of sleepless nights. Nights where I would comfort her and sometimes rock her to sleep in my arms. I continued to do this until she felt safe enough to sleep through the night without waking up screaming or throwing tantrums. I remember some nights just sitting and watching her sleep, stroking her hair, imagining what my life would be like with her long-term.

We bonded more than I had with my first foster child. I was amazed at how her love for me was so pure and innocent. She knew that I would protect her no matter what and did not hold back on showing her appreciation. I now knew what it felt like to have someone love you unconditionally with no strings attached and I loved her just as much. It turns out she had two more younger siblings that I decided to have join us after a few months. This was not a decision that I took lightly. I was passionate, just like my adoptive mom, about keeping the children together, since I too, had been adopted with my two older brothers. I did not want to break up their family bond, so I contacted the caseworker and arranged for them to be placed with me. I was now a single parent, with three toddlers, all three years old and younger. Sound familiar? This was turning out to be the greatest, unexpected adventure I did not know I wanted and needed.

CHAPTER 6
WHEN THEY LEAVE

As previously stated, the main goal of fostering is to reunify the children with their families after a rehabilitation period. This can only happen if they have a family or relatives that want to care for them. If they do not have family or relatives willing to take them in, they become available for adoption. You must go through this cycle if you agree to become a foster parent. I signed up to do this because I had the space in my home, and I had the time to do it, but more importantly, I knew I wanted to be a mom. I already went through the process of losing a child that was not mine, so this should be a piece of cake. Right?

At any time during the fostering period, the juvenile court judge can order the kids to return home. Once the biological family completes the mandated steps on their family plan, the court decides if parents have demonstrated enough progress to have their children returned. If risk at home was decreased during the case, the kids would go back to their loving families, only leaving you with memories if the family does not wish to keep in contact. My job was to take care of them until they could return home, and everything would work out in the end. Surprisingly, this bunch of rowdy kids filling my home with so much love and laughter had me planning a forever with them. I knew, after a few months, I wanted to adopt them. It did not matter that I would probably get stares or side comments for the rest of my life. We were a family, despite our different ethnicities. No one who spent time around us would say different.

It was also during this time, that I started a long-distance relationship with a family friend, who would later become my new husband. After a few months of phone and video chatting, he decided to visit us for a few days. The children fell in love upon meeting him, and he quickly came to accept that if I adopted them, they would be his children too, should we embark upon a long-term relationship. Unfortunately, we would not have the opportunity to adopt these babies because the judge ordered them to return home with their family after sixteen months of being in my care. This was a good thing according to the court system, but it was tragic news for me! With one swift slam of the gavel, my title of "Mommy" became void and my whole family was ripped from me within a couple of hours. Luckily, their family allowed me to visit them at their school and daycare to say my 'good-byes.' Holding them in my arms for the last time as their mother filled me with so much grief and sadness. Heart-wrenching pain barely covers what I felt having to walk away from them one last time. Returning to an empty house to pack up their clothes, toys, and belongings filled me with anger. How could the judge not see that I was the best choice to raise and care for them? How could God not see how much I loved them? Why did I have to go through losing another child? Not just one this time, but three little hearts that I wanted to keep forever. Life was so unfair!

Eventually, I had to face the fact that I was not a mom anymore. I could put away the sippy cups, the giant alphabets we used to learn letters, and turn my children's play area back into an adult space. I had my freedom back. I could find a new routine for all the time I had now. I could finally get back into the gym and start dating exclusively again. I could essentially come and go as I wanted. However, this was a freedom I would gladly give up if only I could get my children back. There were days that I sat and hoped that my phone would ring. That there would be someone on the line saying my kids needed to come back. Hope that the family realized the kids were better off in my care. Unfortunately, this was not realistic, and I had to relearn how to live alone. Again.

If this was how I would feel after every foster child left my care, I did not want to do this again. I could not go through anymore cycles of this type of hurt and pain. I decided to close my home to foster care. I needed a break from loss. My heart was broken, and I was not ready to have another child replace the ones I still sorely missed. I needed a timeout. I tried to find a new rhythm, but the loud silence of the house pushed me into a grief-stricken depression causing me to search for fulfillment elsewhere. I ruined relationships because of selfish choices and turned my back on people who loved me. I tried to smile through it while around others and keep myself busy, but the memories were there waiting for me every time I returned home. I started to see a therapist, but then she quit on me and disappeared too. I could not take it anymore. The sadness and guilt had me running from myself as if I was a fugitive. Eventually, it caught up to me, and I could not bear to face it. I turned my whole life upside down to get away from that emptiness. I packed up my hope, my house, and my life, and finally returned to my home state after almost 11 years. Once again, leaving behind the looming sadness, the memories, and all the mistakes I made in my attempts to find happiness. I was desperate to find my new happy place.

CHAPTER 7
WHO WILL LOVE ME NOW?

Starting over again, *I* felt like a scared foster child. Being uprooted from the life I knew for the last 11 years to go to a familiar but strange place. Yes, I was returning home to family, but I was a different person. I had suffered loss and mental abuse that left emotional scars. I had been through a few heartbreaks and devastations that had changed my life forever. I was not the same woman who went out into the world full of optimism. The woman I saw in the mirror now was one who was fighting to find her place in life again. Struggling to recover the pieces of herself she had given away to those that had said they cared about her. Returning home, I didn't have any choice except to bravely embrace this new season in my life. I had to find out how to fight to become my whole self again. And then put it into action because the pieces of my life were barely hanging on. But I had to move forward.

I had started a long-distance relationship with the man mentioned briefly in the last chapter. In fact, when he could see I was having a hard time and needed a new start, he literally came to get me from Texas and moved me back home to Virginia. We both knew that me coming back home allowed us to see if this relationship could work now that we were in the same state. But I can admit that the thought of going into another serious relationship was scary. Entering with the possibility that I could be the one suffering from infertility issues was even scarier, to say the least. Knowing that I would already have children that he could claim as his own had given me some sense of relief and hope until they were taken away. The great news from my previous primary care provider was that I was fully capable of bearing children. And I was still holding on to that report. However, with no success in my first marriage, I did not want to deprive another husband of leaving a legacy. Yes, I was ahead of myself because marriage was not up for discussion yet, but I wanted to be mentally prepared if he desired to conceive his own children more than he wanted to start a life with me. Could he really be happy if it was just me and him? Would he leave if I could not ultimately bear children?

This was not the case at all. We dated for a little less than a year before we moved in together. Now, this next step was huge for the both of us. After we committed to one another and decided to share a home, I had become restless in waiting for him to make the next move, so I spent a few months fasting and praying for God to fill the longing in my heart, to shift my focus, and to strengthen my relationship with Him. I was so at peace, that I found myself content in being single. Of course, I desired to be married, but when I realized that I would be just fine if him and I went our separate ways, I knew then that I had finally healed. Little did I know, God was working on him as well. Before finding Christ, he was in no hurry to marry and thought he would do so when he decided he was ready. However, God was working on us individually and had other plans for our future together. He surprised me with a marriage proposal that same year, the day after Christmas. I can say with all honesty that I did not see it coming and was shocked to find out he had been working on this for months. We were married less than 40 days later, on my husband's favorite holiday, Superbowl Sunday. Was I truly ready for marriage this time around? I can answer with a resounding YES! My heart was ready to accept him as he was but also be his cheerleader when he was ready to move forward in what God had for him. And he had already proven that he would do the same for me. I genuinely knew that my joy and happiness was not built around him and was confident that our relationship had been ordained by God.

I was again filled with hope for the future knowing that I was married to someone I could envision raising children with. Getting a second chance to create a family with the man I loved was more than I could imagine would happen to me. Therefore, to have to tell your new husband that you have a 10% chance of getting pregnant on your own is devastating. It is not something that he should have to hear, just as much as I did not want to hear it come from the gynecologist. I went in to discuss beginning a family plan and wanted to make sure nothing would prevent me from having a baby this time. After completing labs and ultrasound, this news was not the good news I was expecting. I was finally diagnosed with Endometrial Adenomyosis, which was the cause of me not getting pregnant or being able to maintain a pregnancy after conception. This diagnosis was attributed with Polycystic Ovary Syndrome or PCOS, but it also meant my chances of conceiving on my own were slim to none. My body was not producing enough hormones or making eggs normally, and I was carrying too much weight. I explained this to my husband, not knowing if he would understand that this was beyond my control. He understood that it was not my fault, but this still did not erase the fact that he came into this marriage expecting to have children. Resentment settled in after learning that seeing a fertility specialist, paying thousands of dollars, and going through the treatments was not a guarantee that we would birth children. All of the odds were stacked against me.

To be clear, the resentment he had, was towards the situation, not towards me as his wife. However, I felt guilty, as if I had trapped him in a hopeless situation. I was walking on eggshells for over a week after giving him the news because his initial response was abbreviated. I knew that he needed time to process the news, so I tried not to pressure him into another hard conversation until he was ready. It was a sensitive situation that deserved time to ponder over, and this was his chance to decide whether he would stay or leave. We were only a few months into our first year of marriage and I did not want him to feel obligated to stay with me knowing I could not bear his children. All his friends and family had kids, which made it harder to acknowledge that he may not ever have that opportunity. Furthermore, if we wanted to give conception through In-Vitro Fertilization a fair chance, we would have to break the bank. We were not in any position to do that in the first year of marriage. To afford that process, we would need to actually save the money first and then find a location that we trusted to take us through the process.

This was a pivotal moment in our marriage. My husband and I talked; ultimately deciding that God would have to handle this if we were going to have children naturally. He simply told me that, "God may have wanted it this way" and that "adoption may be the answer for us." Yet again, we were still moving in faith and increasing our intimacy. It did not hurt to keep practicing, and we wanted to give it our best shot. In the meantime, he decided to move forward towards pursuing adoption. The first step would be for him to officially enter the world of foster care to see if this would be a good fit for him. He admitted that he feared the unknown. Not knowing what type of trauma the kids have gone through and not wanting to damage them further. With children coming from different personalities, ethnicities, and backgrounds, all of these could produce a different outcome. Because he has a heart for children, he wanted to be the best foster dad possible. By this time, I had already decided to get back into foster care, so we were currently caring for a pre-teen in our home. Because my husband was not a trained licensed foster parent, he had minimal knowledge of what was and was not acceptable. This strained the relationship between him and our pre-teen so he quickly signed up for the training and went through the classes to learn more about becoming a foster parent who could transition into adoption. Once he completed that training, we added another pre-teen to our home to see if it would be a good fit for all of us. Older children were not our first choice because we were both more comfortable with smaller children, but we had decided to give it a chance.

This was certainly a test for us because the world shut down shortly after his arrival due to an airborne viral pandemic. Forcing us to spend more time together than we normally would have. It was like God was giving us a front-row seat or a crash course in raising kids without the rest of the world's help or resources. There were some wins, but it was not easy with all the personalities stuck in the house for an extended period. In fact, the movie, Instant Family with Mark Wahlberg, gives a great depiction of what it is like entering into the world of Foster Care and Adoption. Others may disagree, but I related to several scenarios from the movie and could feel the new foster mom's frustration. There were some variances for us, but eventually, the children decided they did not want to abide by the rules of the house, so we lovingly let them go. We could have disregarded their feelings, but we wanted children who also wanted us. Although it was a mutual split, we were still sad about them leaving our home because that meant we had not found our forever children. This left us back at square one.

CHAPTER 8
HOUSE OF REFUGE

As of today, we are still in pursuit of our forever children but are choosing to enjoy the journey. We took a break after the pre-teens left to concentrate on strengthening our marriage relationship for a few months. This was important because couples can sometimes lose themselves, their intimacy, and identity as husband and wife when children are in the center of their relationship. Not saying that having children is the issue, but it is vital to remain connected and grounded to one another. Ensuring that the marriage does not become a second or third priority. This also strengthens the stability of the home, giving it a solid foundation to build the family upon.

Looking back, my husband's advice to other men with wives who have a struggle with infertility would be to make sure that you are present for your partner. Make sure that you show up despite how you feel. Should you decide to stay regardless of the diagnosis, pray together for peace, clarity, and wisdom in making decisions that will affect you both. Even though it can be a frustrating time, be sure to comfort your partner and keep them encouraged. Let them know that in the end, everything will be okay. More importantly, do not stop being intimate as this could come off as a sign of rejection. Infertility is a very delicate matter that can affect a man and a woman differently. If left unattended or unacknowledged it could lead to playing the blame game or seeking comfort from others outside of the relationship. This would be detrimental to the entire state of the relationship, not just the area of conception.

My advice to the women would be to first, feel the situation. Pray and seek God for direction, but also have your pity party. Let the tears flow, eat your pint of ice cream, and do whatever it is you need to do, to grieve the unborn children you may never have. Do not try to be Superwoman and skip over that part because you will have to face it at some point. You would rather it be on your terms, than at some friend's baby shower, or in the middle of the supermarket, or when your partner is processing their feelings and needing you to be there for them. Face the situation head-on. Do not stuff your feelings into a corner in the back of your mind. Acknowledge the hurt, disappointment, shame, anger, and whatever emotions that may arise, so that you can heal and move on. Secondly, do not stay there. Do not unpack and live-in pity party land as this will delay the next step in the plan that God has for you. There is a plan to bless you with the children that you are supposed to have. You must be receptive and open to other options to create your family, but you also must be wholly healed to be the best mom possible.

My advice to anyone suffering from infertility issues would be to also look at the big picture. Whether married or single, just know that infertility is not the end of the world. I do not make light of or skim over the huge arena of infertility as it affects thousands of women and the men who love them, including myself. There are many avenues you can explore when trying to start a family so do your research. Do not suffer in silence. Seek out support groups, talk to other people battling the same issue, find what will work best for you. IVF may not be a viable option for everyone due to financial obligations. However, there is also the option of choosing a surrogate to carry the child for you. I, personally, recommend foster care as the best option or a middle ground if you are unsure if adoption or any of these choices are the best routes. Having been through the foster and adoption system myself, I am a product of what happens when someone chooses you.

My life events ultimately prepared me for this journey. If I had not been removed from my biological parents, maybe I would not have grown up with the strength to one day face this same battle my adoptive mother did. I can relate to each kid and together, my husband and I, can push them to be their best selves. We realize, that even though we may not birth our forever children, we can still have a positive influence on any child that comes through our home. We know for certain, that when they leave, they will always have a piece of us that goes with them. The desire to conceive naturally will always be there but we now have a sense of peace with knowing it may not happen. Ultimately, we must realize that families are sometimes created and not always birthed.

Now we have opened our home again to two beautiful little girls who fill our lives with so much love and laughter. They rekindled our love for children and have selfishly stolen our hearts. But we don't mind at all. In fact, we have allowed them free reign when it comes to how much love and affection we share in our home. Recently, following God's guidance, I left the job I had worked for almost three years, essentially cutting our income in half, to stay home to nurture and care for them full time. During this time, my husband and I, have had to sacrifice some things, continue striving to nurture our own relationship, but also, really enjoy just being a family. Our spiritual relationship has deepened with us truly putting our faith and trust in God who has supplied all our needs, plus some. We have seen God's hand at work in keeping us well fed, experienced financial increase, and have not lacked in any area of our life. I believe that God is intentional in His timing and everything He does.

Today, as I sit and watch my two little ones play together, there is a genuine smile on my face as I am enjoying watching them grow, learn, and explore. I choose to love, protect, and nurture them so they can be empowered should they have to leave our care. Their leaving would reset our world again, but I have learned to be content in knowing that the time I have with them is our special time together. Although I am unable to permanently keep every child, a piece of each one stays with me when they leave. That gift helps me to better care for the next one. I urge you to explore the world of foster care because it will immensely change your life. Choosing foster care will either allow you the chance to see if you have the heart to care for someone else's blessing or present you with the opportunity to claim them as your own forever blessings. In whatever age, color, shape, or form they may come, I choose to love all my blessings.